CW00494418

The Ultimate Sirtfood Diet Cookbook for making Desserts and Snacks

50 lovely recipes to enjoy sweet and healthy moments of relax

Anne Patel

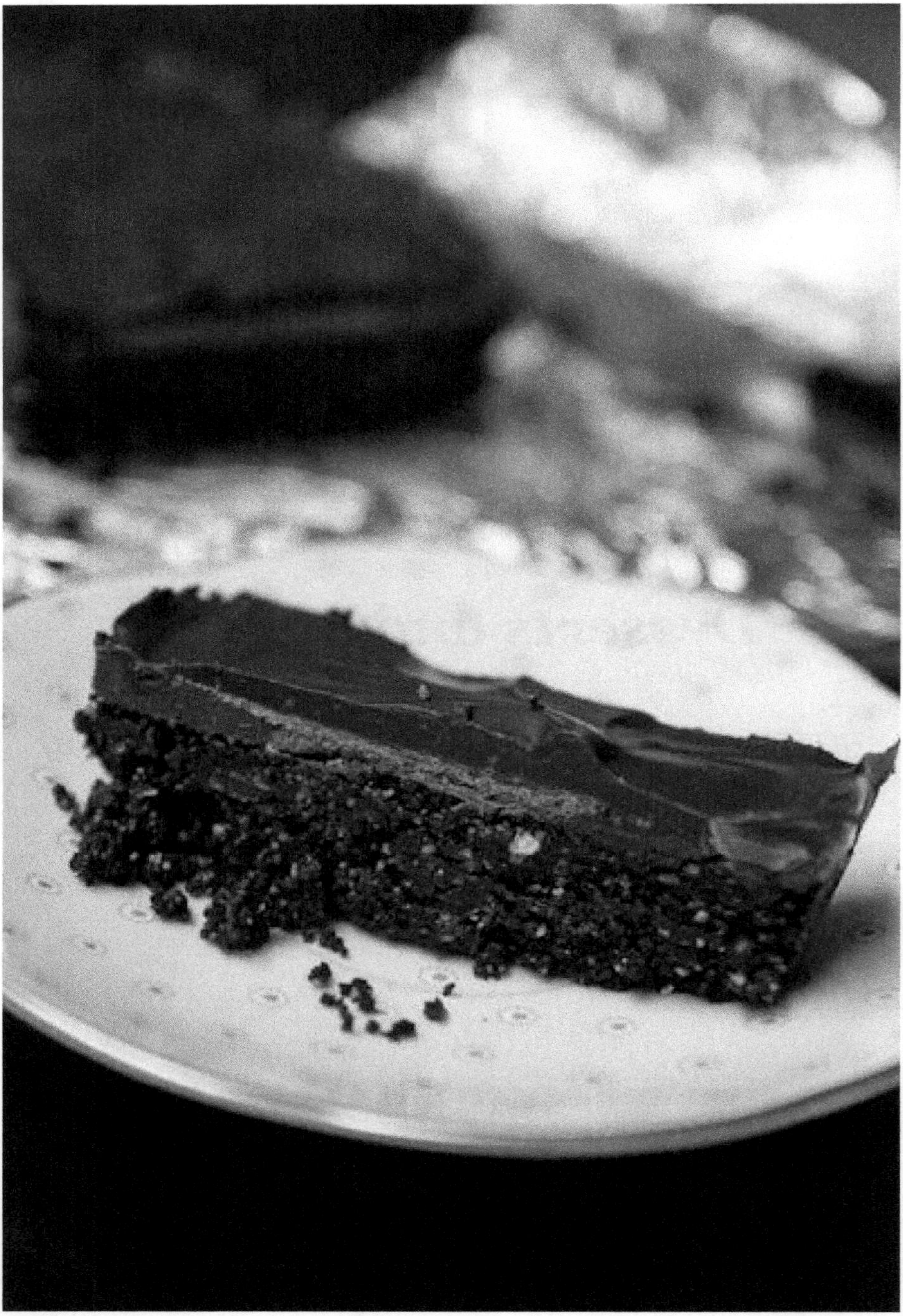

Table of Contents

Chapter 1: What is the Sirtfood diet

The Sirtfood Diet was created by Masters in Nutritional Medicine, Aiden Goggins and Glen Matten.

Their goal initially was to find a healthier way for people to eat, but people started losing weight quickly when they tested their program. With all the people in the world following diets hoping to lose pounds, they thought it would be selfish not to disclose their innovative health plan.

The plan they developed focuses on combining certain foods eaten in order to maximize the supply of nutrition to our body. There is an initial phase in which calories are limited to give the body a period to recover and eliminate accumulated waste. A maintenance phase follows this first phase to accustom the metabolism to the new foods you are ingesting. Throughout all stages, you will incorporate potent green juices and well-structured, well-planned meals.

The diet focuses on so-called 'sirtfoods,' plant-based foods that are known to stimulate a gene called sirtuin in the human body.

Sirtuins belong to an entire protein family, called SIRT1 to SIRT7, and each has specific health-related connections. These proteins help separate and safeguard our cells from inflammation and other damage resulting from everyday activities, helping to reduce our risk of developing major diseases, particularly those related to aging.

Studies have shown that people live longer and healthier lives when they eat diets rich in these foods that activate sirtuin, free from diabetes, heart disease, and even dementia. So this diet was designed to restore a healthy body situation, and one of the byproducts of a healthy body is also the loss of excess weight.

The diet Sirtfood is neither a miracle cure nor a week-long program designed to quickly lose weight before beach holidays. If you are only interested in losing a few pounds and then returning to your old habits, there are certainly plans and diets that are more suited to your needs.

The Sirtfood diet is a project born to help you for the rest of your life, using delicious foods, but that will also improve your health. If you switch from a standard American diet (SAD) to a sirtfood diet, you will lose all the weight your body does not need.

A healthy body does not store extra energy. It asks for what it needs and uses it effectively.

The diet isn't designed to encourage you to starve or deprive yourself. The fact is, foods that are deficient in nutrients are designer made to deprive you and, though the calories are there in plenty, your cells are still starved for the nutrition to help you thrive. The Sirtfood Diet is the opposite of deprivation and starvation. It is nourishment and balance.

Most people following the SAD may use 20 ingredients in a month, let alone enjoy the sheer volume of choice ingredients from the 120 options you will learn about here.

In recent decades, an alarming number of people have come to the conclusion that healthy food is boring, and plants or, more specifically, vegetables are terrible tasting. This is because the foods we've become dependent on – packed with sugar, salt, and unhealthy fats – have chemically altered our connection to food. Our brains are essentially lying to us, and our taste buds have been compromised.

This is one of the reasons the week-long reset is so important. After this first week, you will be able to taste food differently. The more you expose yourself to the recommended plant-based foods, the more pleasure you get out of them.

Sirtuins are critical for our health, regulating many essential biological functions, including our metabolism, which, I'm sure you know, is very closely connected to our weight. It's also a key figure in determining our body composition, such as how much muscle we build and how much fat we retain.

Sirtuin genes regulate all this and more. They're also integral in the process of aging and disease.

If we can turn these genes on, we'll be able to protect our cells and enjoy better health for longer life. Eating sirtfoods is the most effective way to accomplish this goal.

Sirtfoods are all plant-based, and they have many more benefits, in addition to being sirtuin activators.

Our bodies require energy to operate, and the majority of this fuel comes from three primary macronutrients: carbohydrates, fats, and proteins. These macros largely control our metabolic system and regulate how the calories we consume get processed by our bodies. This is why most diets focus exclusively on micronutrition and require you to calculate calories.

Our bodies need more than just energy to survive than thriving, however, which is why micronutrients are so important. They don't impact our weight as obviously as macros, but they are our health foundations.

Micronutrients, such as vitamins, minerals, fiber, antioxidants, and phytonutrients, are supposed to be consumed along with our calories. Unfortunately, in the Standard American Diet (SAD), they're in very limited supply.

When your diet is primarily made up of large quantities of red meat and processed meats, pre-packaged foods, vegetable oils, refined grains and a lot of sugar, you will have an almost total lack of micronutrition.

Plant foods offer the most micronutrients per calorie consumed. Every edible plant has a unique nutritional profile, protecting you from an innumerable variety of illnesses.

Sirtfoods, and other plant-based sources of nutrition, give your body what it needs to stay young and disease-free, and, as a bonus, this will help you remain at an ideal weight.

The original Sirtfood Diet encourages you to commit to a one week reset phase and then a 2-week maintenance phase where you rely heavily on the Sirtfood green juice for a significant dose of nutrition along with meals rich in sirtfoods. Once the phases are complete, to retain your health for the rest of your life, you will need to continue incorporating these sirtfoods into your daily meals.

The Sirtfood Diet is not a miracle cure, but if you stick to these recipes, you'll not just impress your taste buds, but you'll also enhance nearly every aspect of your health. To get safe, you don't have to count calories or starve yourself, the youthful body you've always wanted.

Sirtfood Diet Phases

Every newbie needs to understand that the sirtfood diet does not start with a single list of ingredients in your hands. Its implementation and adaptation are more than mere selective grocery shopping. Every diet can only work effectively when we allow our body to embrace the sudden shift and change in food intake. Similarly, the sirtfood diet also comes with two phases of adaptation. If a dieter successfully goes through these phases, he can continue with the sirtfood diet easily. There are mainly two phases of this diet, which are then succeeded by a third phase in which you can decide how you want to continue the diet.

Phase One

The first seven days of this diet plan are characterized as Phase One. In this phase, a dieter must focus on calorie restriction and the intake of green juices. These seven days are crucial to initiate your weight loss and usually help to lose up to seven pounds if the diet is followed properly. If you find yourself achieving this target, that means that you are on the right track.

In the first three days of the first phase, a dieter must restrict this caloric intake to 1,000 calories only. While doing so, the dieter must also have green juice throughout the day, probably three times a day. Try to drink green juice per meal. The recipes given in the book are perfect for selecting from.

Many meal options can keep your caloric intake in checks, such as buckwheat noodles, seared tofu, some shrimp stir fry, or sirtfood omelet.

Once the first three days of this diet has passed, you can increase your caloric intake to 1,500 calories per day. In these next four days, you can reduce the green juices to two times per side. And pair the juices with more Sirtuin-rich food in every meal.

Phase Two

After the first week of the sirtfood diet, then starts phase two. This phase is more about the maintenance of the diet, as the first week enables the body to embrace the change and start working according to the new diet. This phase enables the body to continue working towards the weight loss objective slowly and steadily. Therefore, the duration of this phase is almost two weeks.

So how is this phase different from phase one? In this phase, there is no restriction on the caloric intake, as long as the food is rich in sirtuins and you are taking it three times a day, it is good to go. Instead of having the green juice two or three times a day, the dieter can have juice one time a day, and that will be enough to achieve steady weight loss. You can have the juice after any meal, in the morning or in the evening.

After the Diet Phase

With the end of phase two comes the time, which is most crucial, and that is the after-diet phase. If your weight loss target has not been reached by the end of step two, then you can restart the phases all over again. Or even when you have achieved the goals but still want to lose more weight, then you can again give it a try.

Instead of following phases one and two over and over again, you can also continue having good quality sirtfood meals in this after-diet phase. Simply continue the eating practices of phase two, have a diet rich in sirtuin and do have green juices whenever possible. The diet is mainly divided into two phases: the first lasts one week, and the other lasts 14 days.

The best 20 sirt foods

All these foods include high quantities of plant compounds called polyphenols, which can be thought to modify the sirtuin enzymes, therefore, excite their super-healthy added benefits.

Top 20 sirtfoods

1. Arugula (Rocket)
2. Buckwheat
3. Capers
4. Celery
5. Chilis
6. Cocoa
7. Coffee
8. Extra Virgin Olive Oil
9. Garlic
10. Green Tea (especially Matcha)
11. Kale
12. Medjool Dates
13. Parsley
14. Red Endive
15. Red Onions
16. Red Wine
17. Soy
18. Strawberries

19. Turmeric
20. Walnuts

What Is So Great About Sirtuins?

There are seven types of Sirtuins named from **SIRT1** to **SIRT7**. Although our understanding of the exact functions of all the Sirtuins is minimal, studies show that activating them can have the following benefits:

Switching on fat burning and protection from weight gain: Sirtuins do this by increasing the mitochondrion's functionality (which is involved in the production of energy) and sparking a change in your metabolism to break down more fat cells.

Improving Memory by protecting neurons from damage. Sirtuins also boost learning skills and memory through the enhancement of synaptic plasticity. Synaptic plasticity refers to synapses' capacity to weaken or strengthen with time due to decreased or increased activity. This is important because memories are represented by different interconnected networks of synapses in the brain, and synaptic plasticity is an important neurochemical foundation of memory and learning.

Slowing down the Ageing Process: Sirtuins act as cell guarding enzymes. Thus, they protect the cells and slow down their aging process.

Repairing cells: The Sirtuins repair cells damaged by re-activating cell functionality.

Protection against diabetes: this happens through prevention against insulin resistance. Sirtuins do this by controlling blood sugar levels because this diet calls for moderate consumption of carbohydrates. These foods cause increases in blood sugar levels; hence the need to release insulin, and as the blood sugar levels increase greatly, there is a need to produce more insulin. Over time, cells become resistant to insulin, hence producing more insulin and leading to insulin resistance.

Fighting Cancers: The chemicals working as sirtuin activators affect the function of sirtuin in different cells, i.e. by switching it on when in normal cells and shutting it down in cancerous cells. This encourages the death of cancerous cells.

Fighting inflammation: Sirtuins have a powerful antioxidant effect that has the power to reduce oxidative stress. This has positive effects on heart health and cardiovascular protection.

Chapter 2: How do the Sirtfood Diet Works?

The basis of the sirtuin diet can be explained in simple terms or in complex ways. However, it's important to understand how and why it works so that you can appreciate the value of what you are doing. It is important to also know why these sirtuin rich foods help to help you maintain fidelity to your diet plan. Otherwise, you may throw something in your meal with less nutrition that would defeat the purpose of planning for one rich in sirtuins. Most importantly, this is not a dietary fad, and as you will see, there is much wisdom contained in how humans have used natural foods, even for medicinal purposes, over thousands of years.

To understand how the Sirtfood diet works and why these particular foods are necessary, we're going to look at their role in the human body.

Sirtuin activity was first researched in yeast, where a mutation caused an extension in the yeast's lifespan. Sirtuins were also shown to slow aging in laboratory mice, fruit flies, and nematodes. As research on Sirtuins proved to transfer to mammals, they were examined for their use in diet and slowing the aging process. The sirtuins in humans are different in typing, but they essentially work in the same ways and reasons.

The Sirtuin family is made up of seven "members." It is believed that sirtuins play a big role in regulating certain functions of cells, including proliferation, reproduction and growth of cells), apoptosis death of cells). They promote survival and resist stress to increase longevity.

They are also seen to block neurodegeneration loss or function of the nerve cells in the brain). They conduct their housekeeping functions by cleaning out toxic proteins and supporting the brain's ability to change and adapt to different conditions or to recuperate i.e., brain plasticity). They also help minimize chronic inflammation as part of this and decrease anything called oxidative stress. Oxidative stress is when there are so many free radicals present in the body that are cell-damaging, and by fighting them with antioxidants, the body can not keep up. These factors are related to age-related illness and weight as well, which again brings us back to a discussion of how they actually work.

You will see labels in Sirtuins that start with "SIR," which represents "Silence Information Regulator" genes. They do exactly that, silence or regulate, as part of their functions. Humans work with the seven sirtuins: SIRT1, SIRT2, SIRT3,

SIRT4, SIRT 5, SIRT6 and SIRT7. Each of these types is responsible for different areas of protecting cells. They work by either stimulating or turning on certain gene expressions or by reducing and turning off other gene expressions. This essentially means that they can influence genes to do more or less of something, most of which they are already programmed to do.

Through enzyme reactions, each of the SIRT types affects different areas of cells responsible for the metabolic processes that help maintain life. This is also related to what organs and functions they will affect.

For example, the SIRT6 causes and expression of genes in humans that affect skeletal muscle, fat tissue, brain, and heart. SIRT 3 would cause an expression of genes that affect the kidneys, liver, brain and heart.

If we tie these concepts together, you can see that the Sirtuin proteins can change the expression of genes, and in the case of the Sirtfood diet, we care about how sirtuins can turn off those genes that are responsible for speeding up aging and for weight management.

The other aspect to this conversation of sirtuins is the function and the power of calorie restriction on the human body. Calorie restriction is simply eating fewer calories. This, coupled with exercise and reducing stress, is usually a combination for weight loss. Calorie restriction has also proven across much research in animals and humans to increase one's lifespan.

We can look further at the role of sirtuins with calorie restriction and using the SIRT3 protein, which has a role in metabolism and aging. Amongst all of the effects of the protein on gene expression, such as preventing cells from dying, reducing tumors from growing, etc.), we want to understand the effects of SIRT3 on weight for this book's purpose.

As we stated earlier, the SIRT3 has high expression in those metabolically active tissues, and its ability to express itself increases with caloric restriction, fasting, and exercise. On the contrary, it will express itself less when the body has high fat, high calorie-riddled diet.

The last few highlights of sirtuins are their role in regulating telomeres and reducing inflammation, which also helps with staving off disease and aging.

Telomeres are sequences of proteins at the ends of chromosomes. When cells divide, these get shorter. As we age, they get shorter, and other stressors to the body also will contribute to this. Maintaining these longer telomeres is the key to slower aging. In addition, proper diet, along with exercise and other variables, can lengthen telomeres. SIRT6 is one of the sirtuins that, if activated, can help with DNA damage, inflammation and oxidative stress. SIRT1 also helps with inflammatory response cycles that are related to many age-related diseases.

Calories restriction can extend life to some degree. Since this and fasting are a stressor, these factors will stimulate the SIRT3 proteins to kick in and protect the body from the stressors and excess free radicals. Again, the telomere length is affected as well.

Having laid this all out before you, you should appreciate how and why these miraculous compounds work in your favor, keep you youthful, healthy, and lean If they are working hard for you, don't you feel that you should do something too?

50 Desserts and Snacks Recipes

1. Pear, Cranberry and Chocolate Crisp

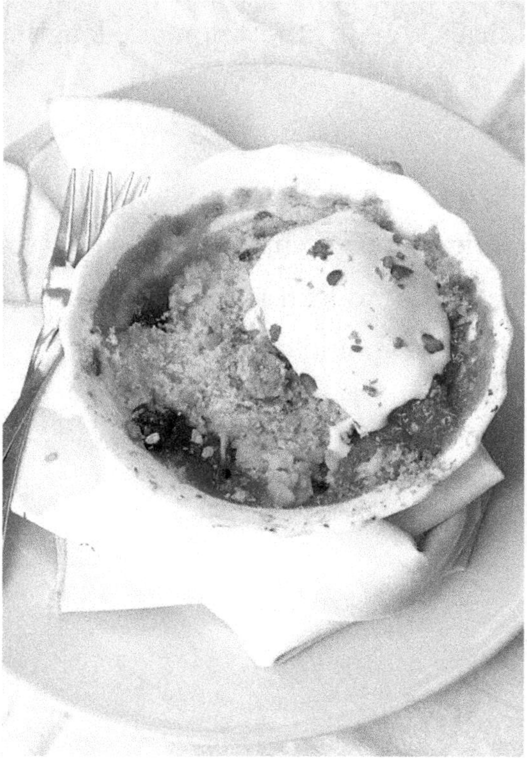

Preparation Time: 15 Minutes

Cooking Time: 10 Minutes

Servings: 10

Ingredients:

1/2 cup flour

1/2 cup brown sugar

1 tsp. cinnamon

1/8 tsp. salt

3/4 cup yogurt

1/4 cup sliced peppers

1/3 cup butter, melted

1 teaspoon vanilla

Filling:

1 tbsp. brown sugar

1/4 cup dried cranberries

1 teaspoon of lemon juice

Two handfuls of milk chocolate chips

Directions:

1. Preheat oven to 375.

2. Using butter spray to spray a casserole dish.

3. Put all of the topping **ingredients** – flour, sugar, cinnamon, salt, nuts, etc.

4. Butter a bowl and then mix. Set aside.

5. Combine the sugar, lemon juice, pears and cranberries in a big cup.

6. Once is fully blended, move to the prepared baking dish.

7. Spread the topping evenly over the fruit.

8. Bake for about half an hour.

9. Disperse chocolate chips out at the top.

10. Cook for another 10 minutes.

11. Have with ice cream.

Nutrition: Calories: 128 Cal Fat: 6.6 g Carbs: 15 g Fiber: 0.7 g Protein: 2 g

2. Radish green pesto

Preparation Time: 15 Minutes
Cooking Time: 60 Minutes
Servings: 10

Ingredients:
2 handfuls
fresh radish leaf (from 1–2 bunch of radishes in organic quality)
1 garlic
30 g pine nuts (2 tbsp)
30 g parmesan (1 piece; 30% fat in dry matter)
100 ml olive oil
salt
pepper
1 tsp lemon juice

Directions:
1. Wash the radish leaves and shake them dry. Peel and chop the garlic.

2. Roast pine nuts in a hot pan without fat over medium heat for 3 minutes. Grate the Parmesan finely.

3. Puree the radish leaves, garlic, pine nuts and the oil with a hand blender. Mix in the Parmesan. Season with salt, pepper and lemon juice.

3. Watercress smoothie

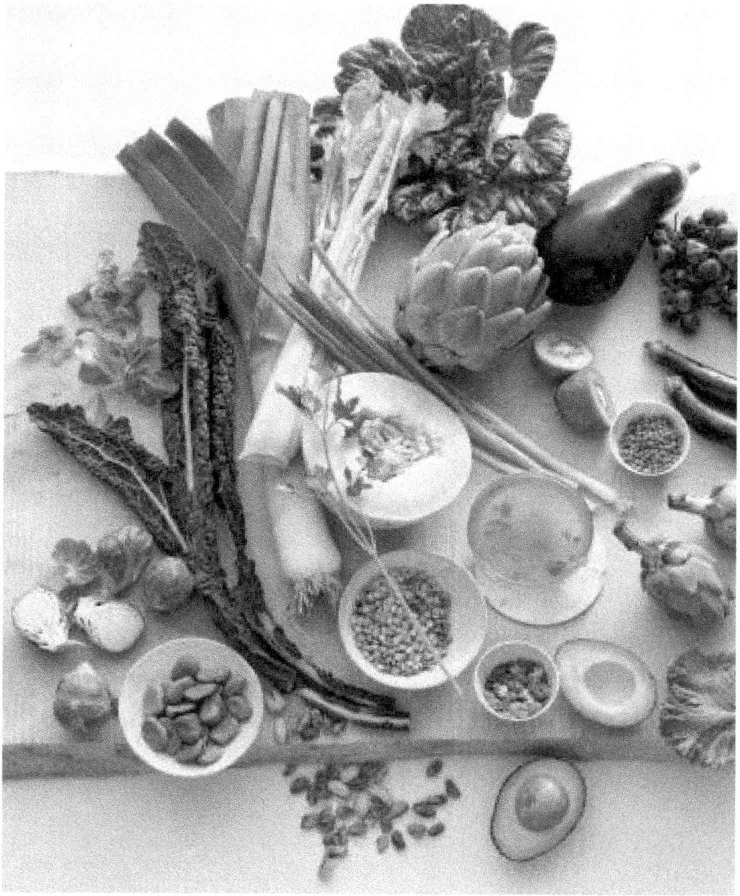

Preparation Time: 15 Minutes

Cooking Time: 60 Minutes

Servings: 10

Ingredients:

150 g watercress

1 small onion

½ cucumber

1 tbsp lemon juice

200 ml mineral water

salt

pepper

4 tbsp crushed ice

Directions:

1. Wash and spin dry watercress; put some sheets aside for the garnish.

2. The onion should be peeled and cut into small cubes. Wash the cucumber half, halve lengthways and cut the pulp into tiny cubes; Set aside 4 tablespoons of cucumber cubes.

3. Puree the remaining cucumber cubes with cress, onion cubes, lemon juice, mineral water and ice in a blender.

4. Season the smoothie with salt and pepper, pour into 2 glasses and sprinkle with cucumber cubes and cress leaves.

4. Melon and spinach juice with cinnamon

Preparation Time: 15 Minutes
Cooking Time: 60 Minutes
Servings: 10

Ingredients:
350 g small honeydew melon (0.5 small honeydew melons)
250 g young tender spinach leaves
1 PC cinnamon stick (approx. 1 cm)
nutmeg

Directions:
1. Core the melon with a teaspoon. First cut the melon into wedges, then cut the pulp from the skin and roughly dice.

2. Clean the spinach and wash thoroughly in a bowl of water. Renew the water several times until it remains clear.

3. Using a small sharp knife, scrape thin strips off the cinnamon stick.

4. Squeeze the spinach lightly; Put back a leaflet and a small stem for the garnish as you like. Juice the rest with the melon in a juicer and pour it into a glass with ice cubes. Rub a little

nutmeg over it, garnish with cinnamon and possibly with the spinach set aside and enjoy immediately.

5. Christmas cocktail - vegan eggnog

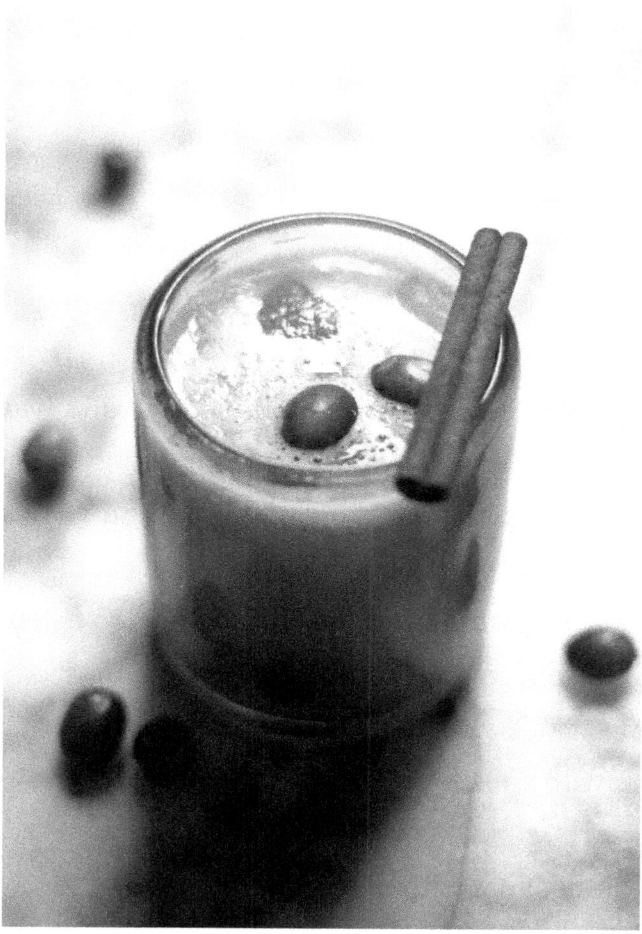

Ingredients

1 cup cashew nuts

1 cup soy or almond milk

2-3 glasses of water

about 5 pieces of dates (more if you like sweeter drinks)

2-3 scoops of brandy or whiskey

1 tablespoon lemon juice (optional, to taste)

1-2 teaspoons cinnamon

½ teaspoons ground anise

½ teaspoons ground ginger

2 pinches nutmeg

pinch of salt

Directions:

1. Pour dates and cashews with boiling water and leave to soak for 20 minutes. Transfer the remaining ingredients to the blender dish and finally add the drained nuts and dates.

2. Mix thoroughly in a high-speed blender for a few minutes, until a thick and creamy cocktail without lumps is formed. If your blender can't do it, mix the cashews with water first and strain them with gauze.

3. Season the cocktail with more lemon juice and salt to tasteand if you prefer sweeter drinks, add 2-3 pieces of dates. Serve it chilled with a pinch of cinnamon.

6. Orange and mandarin liqueur

Preparation Time: 15 Minutes

Cooking Time: 60 Minutes

Servings: 10

Ingredients:

2 large oranges

2 tangerines

1 small lemon

300 g white sugar candy

1 stick of vanilla

50 ml of orange juice

250 ml double grain

Directions:

1. Put the sugar candy in a bottle or a screw-top jar.

2. Pour the citrus into small pieces and remove the skin.

3. Pour in the orange juice.

4. Add the vanilla stick.

5. Baste with the double grain
6. Fill up to the top of the bottle if desired.

7. Close the bottle.

8. Shake daily until the sugar candy has dissolved.

9. After 2 - 3 weeks pour the liqueur through a sieve.

10. Pour it back into the bottle.

7. Cucumber-apple-banana shake

Preparation Time: 15 Minutes
Cooking Time: 60 Minutes
Servings: 10

Ingredients:

1 lemon
1 banana
4th sour apples (e.g. granny smith)
1 bunch parsley
½ cucumber
mineral water to fill up
10 dice ice cubes

Directions:

1. Break the lemon in half and suck the juice out. Peel and dice the banana. Clean, wash, quarter the apples, remove the core, dice the pulp. Mix the apples with the banana cubes and lemon juice.

2. Wash parsley, shake dry and chop. Clean, peel and halve the cucumber, coreand cut into bite-size pieces. Put 3 pieces of cucumber on 4 wooden skewers.

3. Puree the remaining pieces of cucumber with fruit, parsley and ice in a blender. Spread over 4 glasses, fill up with mineral water to the desired consistency and garnish with 1 cucumber skewer each.

8. Kefir avocado shake with herbs

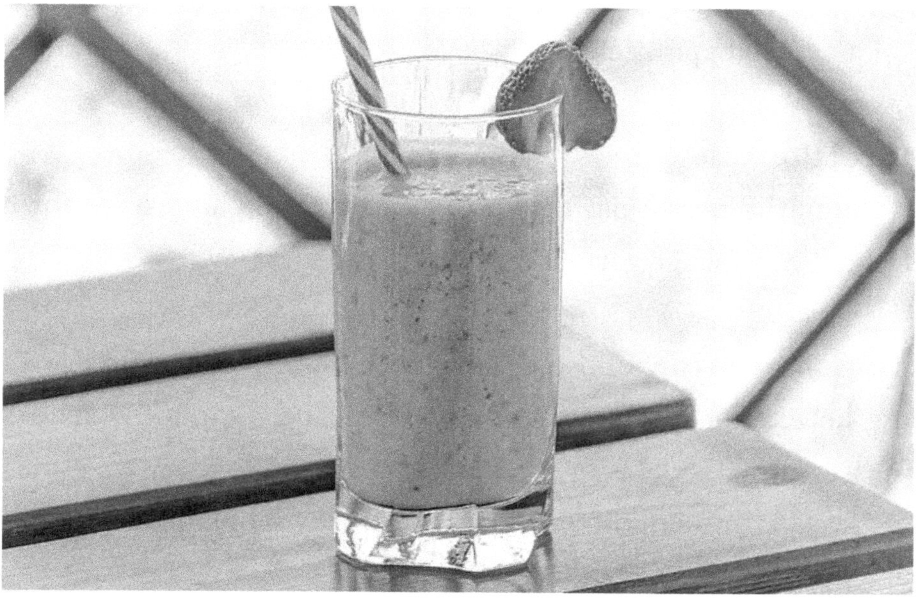

Preparation Time: 15 Minutes

Cooking Time: 60 Minutes

Servings: 10

Ingredients:

2 stems dill

2 stems parsley

straws of chives

1 avocado

1 tsp honey

1 splash lime juice

4 ice cubes

300 ml kefir chilled

salt

1 pinch wasabi powder

Directions:

1. Spray the herbs, pat dry, pluck and cut roughly except for a few dill tips for the garnish.

2. Peel, halve, core and cut the avocado into pieces. Puree with the herbs, honey, lime juice, ice cubes and kefir in a blender until creamy.

3. Season the smoothie with salt and wasabi and pour into glasses. Serve garnished with dill tips.

9. Mandarin liqueur

Preparation Time: 15 Minutes
Cooking Time: 60 Minutes
Servings: 10

Ingredients:
2 large oranges
2 tangerines
1 small lemon
300 g white sugar candy
1 stick of vanilla
50 ml of orange juice
250 ml double grain

Directions:
1. Put the sugar candy in a bottle or a screw-top jar.

2. Pour the citrus into small pieces and remove the skin.

3. Pour in the orange juice.

4. Add the vanilla stick.

5. Baste with the double grain and fill up to the top of the bottle if desired.

6. Close the bottle.

7. Shake daily until the sugar candy has dissolved.

8. After 2 - 3 weeks pour the liqueur through a sieve and pour it back into the bottle.

10. Pear and lime marmalade

Ingredients for 1.5 l jam

3-4 untreated limes

1 kg ripe pears

500 g jam sugar 2: 1

Directions:

1. Wash 2 limes and grate dry.

2. Peel the peels thinly with the zest ripper.

3. Then cut all limes in half and squeeze them out. Measure out100 ml of lime juice.

4. Wash and peel the pears, remove the core and then quarter them. Weigh 900 g of pulp.

5. Then puree the pears together with the lime juice.

6. Now put the pear puree together with the lime peels and the jellied sugar in a saucepan.

7. Bring all **ingredients** to the boil together.

8. Simmer for 4 minutes, stirring, taking care not to burn anything.

9. Make a gelation test with a small blob on a cold saucer. If this becomes solid in a short time, the jam is ready.

10. Remove any foam that may have formed with a spade, but you can also simply stir it in.

11. Then pour the hot mass into hot rinsed jars, close and let stand upside down.

11. Healthy green shot

Preparation Time: 15 Minutes

Cooking Time: 60 Minutes

Servings: 10

Ingredients:

2 pears

3 green apples (e.g. granny smith)

3 sticks celery

60 g organic ginger

1 bunch parsley (20 g)

3 kiwi fruit

2 limes

1 tsp turmeric

Directions:

1. Wash pears, apples, celery, ginger and parsley and cut into pieces. Halve the kiwi fruit and remove the pulp with a spoon. Halve limes and squeeze out juice.

2. Put the pears, apples, kiwi, celery, ginger and parsley in the juicer and squeeze out the juice.

3. Mix freshly squeezed juice with the lime juice and season with turmeric. Serve the mixture as shots immediately or freeze it in portions.

12. Spinach kiwi smoothie bowl

Preparation Time: 15 Minutes
Cooking Time: 60 Minutes
Servings: 10

Ingredients:
1 green apple
2 kiwi fruit
300 g bananas (2 bananas)
100 g baby spinach
1 lemon
6 g chia seeds (2 tsp)
20 g grated coconut (2 tbsp)

Directions:
1. Clean, wash, core and chop the apple. Peel and cut the kiwis and bananas and put half aside. Wash the spinach and put some leaves aside. Halve the lemon and squeeze out the juice.

2. Put half of the fruit, spinach and lemon juice in a blender and mash finely. Divide the smoothie into 4 bowls.

3. Put the remaining pieces of fruit as a topping on the smoothie bowls. Sprinkle with chia seeds and grated coconut and serve with the remaining spinach leaves.

13. Avocado smoothie with basil

Preparation Time: 15 Minutes
Cooking Time: 60 Minutes
Servings: 10

Ingredients:
2 kiwi fruit
1 yellow-peeled apple
200 g honeydew melon meat
1 avocado
1 green chili pepper
20 g basil (1 handful)
20 g arugula (0.25 bunch)
1 tbsp sprouts (suitable for raw consumption)

Directions:
1. Peel and slice the kiwi fruit. Clean the apple, quarter and core it and break the quarters into slices. Cut the melon meat into pieces. Peel, core and cut avocado into pieces. Wash the chili pepper and cut it into rings. Wash the basil and rocket and shake dry. Shower sprouts in a sieve.

2. Put all prepared **ingredients** in a blender and mash them finely. Add about 100 ml of cold water and serve in 4 glasses.

14. Blackberry and vanilla smoothie

Preparation Time: 15 Minutes
Cooking Time: 60 Minutes
Servings: 10

Ingredients:
500 g blackberry
1 vanilla bean
1 tsp lemon juice
700 ml buttermilk (ice cold)
80 g lean quark (4 tbsp)
40 g cashews
80 ml whipped cream

Directions:
1. Wash and drain blackberries.

2. Cut the length of the vanilla pod, scrape the creamy pulp and puree in a blender with blackberries, lemon juice, buttermilk, curd cheese and cashew nuts.

3. Whip the cream. Pour smoothie into 4 glasses and garnish with cream

15. Dijon Celery Salad

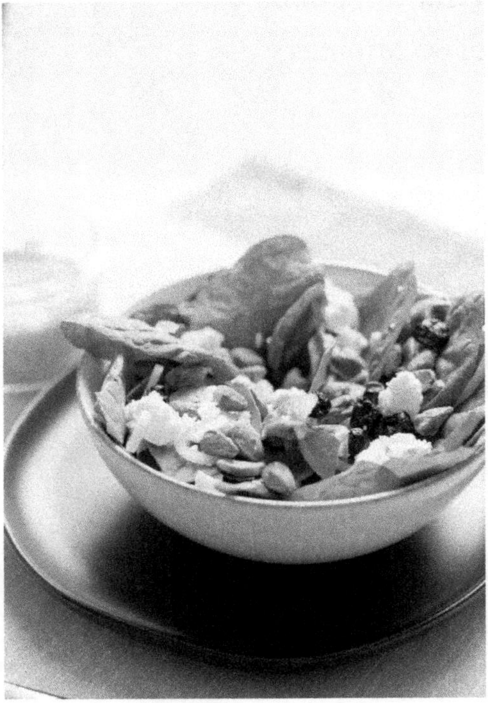

Preparation Time: 10 minutes

Cooking Time: 0 minutes

Servings: 4

Ingredients:

5 teaspoons stevia

½ cup lemon juice

1/3 cup dijon mustard

2/3 cup olive oil

black pepper to the taste

2 apples, cored, peeled and cubed

1 bunch celery and leaves, roughly chopped ¾ cup walnuts, chopped

Directions:

1. In a salad bowl, mix celery and its leaves with apple pieces and walnuts.

2. Add black pepper, lemon juice, mustard, stevia and olive oil.

3. Whisk well, add to your salad, toss.

4. Divide into small cups and serve as a snack.

Nutrition: Calories: 125 Cal Fat: 2 g Carbohydrates: 7 g Protein: 7 g Fiber: 2 g

16. Dill Bell Pepper Snack Bowls

Preparation Time: 10 minutes

Cooking Time: 0 minutes

Servings: 4

Ingredients:

2 tablespoons dill, chopped

1 yellow onion, chopped

1-pound multicolored bell peppers, cut into halves, seeded and cut into thin strips

3 tablespoons olive oil

2 and ½ tablespoons white vinegar

Black pepper to the taste

Directions:

1. In a salad bowl, mix bell peppers with onion, dill, pepper, oil and vinegar, toss to coat, divide into small bowls and serve as a snack.

Nutrition: Calories: 120 Cal Fat: 3 g Carbohydrates: 2 g Protein: 3 g Fiber: 3 g

17. Cinnamon Apple Chips

Preparation Time: 10 minutes

Cooking Time: 2 hours

Servings: 4

Ingredients:

Cooking spray

2 teaspoons cinnamon powder

2 apples, cored and thinly sliced

Directions:

On a lined baking sheet, arrange the apple slices, sprinkle with cooking oil, sprinkle with cinnamon, place in the oven and cook at 300 degrees F for 2 hours.

Divide and serve as a snack in bowls.

Nutrition: Calories: 80 Cal Fat: 0 g Carbohydrates: 7 g Protein: 4 g Fiber: 3 g

18. Herb Roasted Chickpeas

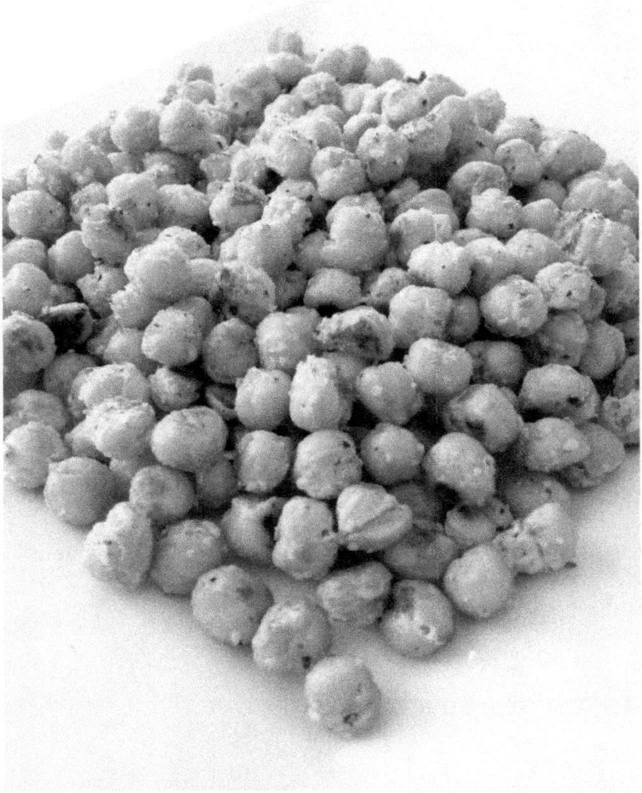

Preparation time: 5 minutes

Cooking time: 30 minutes

Servings: 3

Ingredients:

1 can of chickpeas, drained

1 - 2 tablespoon extra-virgin olive oil

½ teaspoon dried lovage

½ teaspoon dried basil

1 teaspoon garlic powder

1/8 teaspoon cayenne powder

¼ teaspoon fine salt

Directions:

Preheat the oven to 400 degrees F and use parchment paper to cover a large baking sheet.

Spread chickpeas out evenly over the pan in a single layer and roast for 30 minutes.

Remove from oven and transfer to a heat-resistant bowl.

Add the olive oil and toss to coat each chickpea. Sprinkle with herbs and toss again to distribute.

Return to oven for an additional 15 minutes.

Until eating, let it cool for at least 15 minutes.

19. Beans Snack Salad

Preparation Time: 10 minutes

Cooking Time: 0 minutes

Servings: 6

Ingredients:

2 cups tomatoes, chopped

2 cups cucumber, chopped

3 cups mixed greens

2 cups mung beans, sprouted

2 cups clover sprouts

for the salad dressing:

1 tablespoon cumin, ground

1 cup dill, chopped

4 TABLESPOONS LEMON JUICE

1 avocado, pitted, peeled and roughly chopped

1 cucumber, roughly chopped

Directions:

1. In a salad bowl.

2. Mix tomatoes with 2 cups cucumber, greens, clover and mung sprouts.

3. In your blender, mix cumin with dill, lemon juice, 1 cucumber and avocado.

4. Blend well, add this to your salad, toss well and serve as a snack.

Nutrition: Calories: 120 Cal Fat: 0 g Carbohydrates: 1 g Protein: 6 g Fiber: 2 g

20. Sprouts and Apple Snack Salad

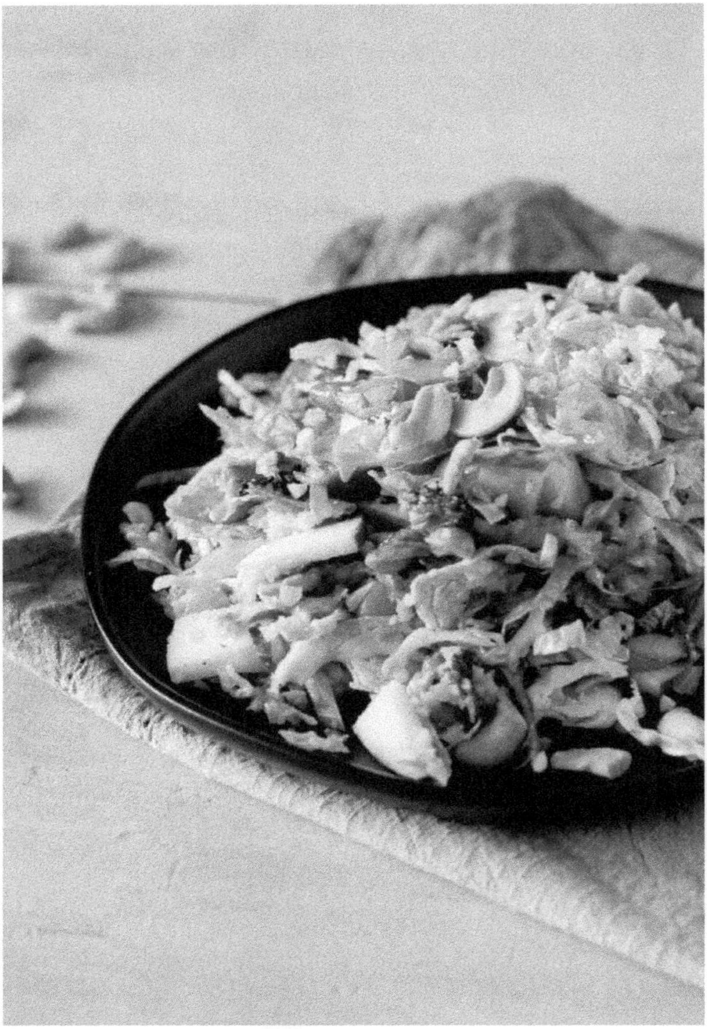

Preparation Time: 10 minutes

Cooking Time: 0 minute

Servings: 4

Ingredients:

1-pound brussels sprouts, shredded

1 cup walnuts, chopped

1 apple, cored and cubed

1 red onion, chopped

For the salad dressing:

3 tablespoons red vinegar

1 tablespoon mustard

1/2 cup olive oil

1 garlic clove, minced

Black pepper to the taste

Directions:

1. In a salad bowl, mix sprouts with apple, onion and walnuts.

2. In another bowl, mix vinegar with mustard, oil, garlic and pepper, whisk well, add this to your salad, toss well and serve as a snack.

Nutrition: Calories: 120 Cal Fat: 2 g Carbohydrates: 8 g Protein: 6 g Fiber: 2 g

21. Celery and Raisins Snack Salad

Preparation Time: 10 minutes

Cooking Time: 0 minutes

Servings: 4

Ingredients:

½ cup raisins

4 cups celery, sliced

¼ cup parsley, chopped

½ cup walnuts, chopped

Juice of ½ lemon

2 tablespoons olive oil

Salt and black pepper to the taste

Directions:

1. In a salad bowl.

2. Mix celery with raisins, walnuts, parsley, lemon juice, oil and black pepper, toss

3. Divide into small cups and serve as a snack.

Nutrition: Calories: 120 Cal Fat: 1 g Carbohydrates: 6 g Protein: 5 g Fiber: 2 g

22. Mozzarella Bars

Preparation Time: 10 minutes
Cooking Time: 40 minutes
Servings: 12

Ingredients:
1 big cauliflower head, riced
½ cup low-fat mozzarella cheese, shredded
¼ cup egg whites
1 teaspoon Italian seasoning
Black pepper to the taste

Directions:
1. Spread the cauliflower rice on a lined baking sheet, cook in the oven at 375 degrees F for 20 minutes.

2. Transfer to a bowl, add black pepper, cheese, seasoning and egg whites.

3. Stir well, spread into a rectangle pan and press on the bottom.

4. Introduce in the oven at 375 degrees F, bake for 20 minutes, cut into 12 bars.

5. and serve as a snack.

Nutrition: Calories: 140 Cal Fat: 1 g Carbohydrates: 6 g Protein: 6 g Fiber: 3 g

23. Eggplant Salsa

Preparation Time: 10 minutes
Cooking Time: 10 minutes
Servings: 4

Ingredients:
1 AND ½ CUPS TOMATOES, CHOPPED
3 cups eggplant, cubed
a drizzle of olive oil
2 teaspoons capers
6 ounces green olives, pitted and sliced
4 garlic cloves, minced
2 teaspoons balsamic vinegar
1 tablespoon basil, chopped
black pepper to the taste

Directions:
1. Heat a pan with the oil over medium-high heat, add eggplant, stirand cook for 5 minutes. Add tomatoes, capers, olives, garlic, vinegar, basil and black pepper, toss, cook for 5 minutes more, divide into small cupsand serve cold.

Nutrition: Calories: 120 Cal Fat: 6 g Carbohydrates: 9 g Protein: 7 g Fiber: 5 g

24. Date Nut Bread

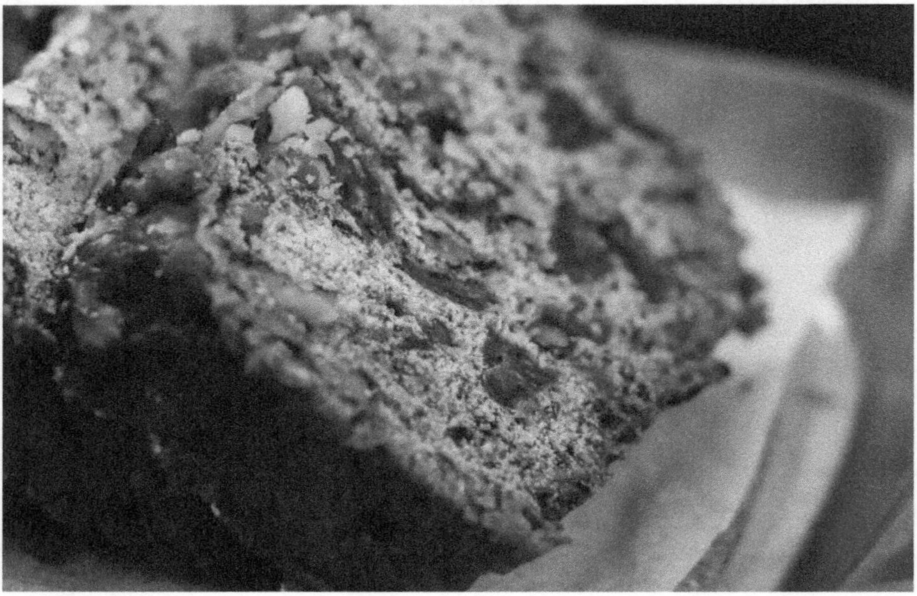

Preparation Time: 30 minutes

Cooking Time: 4-6 hours

Servings: 4-6

Ingredients:

¾ cup Medjool dates

1 ¼ cup All-Purpose flour

2 teaspoon baking powder

¼ teaspoon baking soda

½ teaspoon salt

½ cup sugar

¾ cup milk

1 egg, slightly beaten

1 tablespoon orange peel, grated

1 tablespoon coconut oil, melted

¼ cup buckwheat flour

1 cup walnuts, chopped

Directions:

1. On a chopping board, put the dates and sprinkle 1 tablespoon of All-Purpose flour over them. Dip a knife into the flour and finely chop the dates. Flour the knife sometimes to avoid sticking the cut-up fruit together.
2. Sift the remaining All-Purpose flour, baking powder, baking soda, salt and sugar into a large bowl.

3. Combine the milk, egg, orange peel and oil in a separate dish.

4. Add the buckwheat flour to the flour mixture, mix well and gently fold in the dates, along with any flour left on the cutting block and the walnuts.

5. Pour in the liquid **ingredients** and mix until just combined.

6. Transfer dough into a well-greased and floured baking unit. Cover and place in the slow cooker

7. Use a toothpick or small amount of twisted aluminum foil to prop the crockpot lid open a tiny fraction to allow steam to escape.

8. Cook on high for 4 to 6 hours. Cool on a rack for 10 minutes. Serve warm or cold.

9. Do NOT lift the crockpot lid while the bread is baking.

Nutrition: Calories: 70 Cal Fat:1 g Carbohydrates: 15 g Protein: 1 g Fiber: 1 g

25. Strawberry Rhubarb Crisp

Preparation Time: 10 minutes

Cooking Time: 45 minutes

Servings: 6-8

Ingredients:

1 cup white sugar

½ cup buckwheat flour + 3 tablespoons

3 cups strawberries, sliced

3 cups rhubarb, diced

½ lemon, juiced

1 cup packed brown sugar

1 cup coconut oil, melted

¾ cup rolled oats

¼ cup buckwheat groats

¼ cup walnuts, chopped

Directions:

1. Preheat oven to 375 degrees F

2. Combine the white sugar, 3 tablespoons of flour, strawberries, rhubarb, and lemon juice in a large bowl. Place a 9x13 inch baking dish with the mixture.

3. Mix 1/2 cup of flour, brown sugar, coconut oil, oats, buckwheat grits and walnuts in a separate bowl until crumbly. For this, you may wish to use a pastry blender. Crumble the rhubarb and strawberry mixture on top.

4. Bake in a preheated oven for 45 minutes, or until crisp and lightly browned.

Nutrition: Calories: 240 Cal Fat: 7 g Carbohydrates: 42 g Protein: 2 g Fiber: 3 g

26. Veggie Cakes

Preparation Time: 30 Minutes
Cooking Time: 30 Minutes
Servings: 8

INGREDIENTS:

Two teaspoons ginger, grated
1 cup yellow onion, chopped
1 cup mushrooms, minced
1 cup canned red lentils, drained
¼ cup veggie stock
One sweet potato, chopped
¼ cup parsley, chopped
¼ cup hemp seeds
One tablespoon curry powder
¼ cup cilantro, chopped
A drizzle of olive oil
1 cup quick oats
Two tablespoons rice flour

DIRECTIONS:

1. Warmth a pan with the oil on medium-high heat, add ginger, onion, and mushrooms, stir, and cook for 2-3 minutes.

2. Add lentils, potato, and stock, stir, cook for 5-6 minutes, take off heat, cool the whole mixture, and mash it with a fork.

3. Add parsley, cilantro, hemp, oats, curry powder, and rice flour, stir well and shape medium cakes out of this mix.

4. Place veggie cakes in your air fryer's basket and cook at 3750 F for 10 minutes, flipping them halfway.

5. Serve them as an appetizer.

NUTRITION: Calories: 212 Fat: 4 grams Net Carbs: 8 grams Protein: 10 grams

27. Cinnamon Coconut Chips

Preparation Time: 7 Minutes

Cooking Time: 25 Minutes

Servings: 2

INGREDIENTS:

¼ cup coconut chips, unsweetened

¼ teaspoon of sea salt

¼ cup cinnamon

DIRECTIONS:

1. Add cinnamon and salt in a mixing bowl and set aside. Heat a pan over medium heat for 2 minutes.

2. Place the coconut chips in the hot pan and stir until coconut chips crisp and lightly brown.

3. Toss toasted coconut chips with cinnamon and salt.

NUTRITION: Calories: 228 Fat: 21 grams Net Carbs: 7.8 grams Protein: 1.9 grams

28. Peach Cobbler

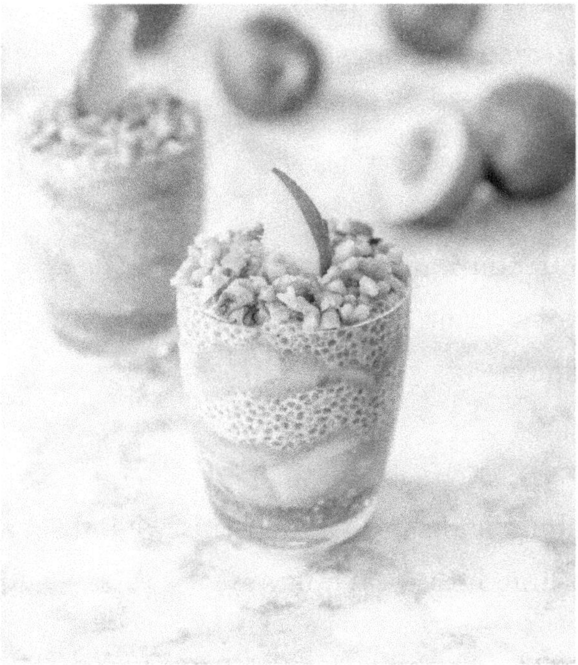

Preparation Time: 20 Minutes

Cooking Time: 4 hours

Servings: 4

INGREDIENTS:

4 cups peaches, peeled and sliced

¼ cup of coconut sugar

½ teaspoon cinnamon powder

1 ½ cups vegan sweet crackers, crushed ¼ cup stevia

¼ teaspoon nutmeg, ground
½ cup almond milk
One teaspoon vanilla extract
Cooking spray

DIRECTIONS:

1. In a bowl, mix peaches with coconut sugar and cinnamon and stir.

2. In a separate bowl, mix crackers with stevia, nutmeg, almond milk, and vanilla extract and stir.

3. Shower your slow cooker with cooking spray and spread peaches on the bottom.

4. Add crackers mix, spread, cover, and cook on Low for 4 hours.

5. Divide cobbler between plates and serve.

NUTRITION: Calories: 212 Fat: 4 grams Net Carbs: 7 grams Protein: 3 grams

29. Chocolate Brownies

Preparation Time: 10 Minutes

Cooking Time: 20 Minutes

Servings: 4

INGREDIENTS:

Two tablespoons cocoa powder

One scoop protein powder

1 cup bananas, over-ripe

½ cup almond butter, melted

DIRECTIONS:

1. Preheat the oven to 3500 F.

2. Spray the brownie pan with cooking spray.

3. Add the real ingredients in your blender and blend until smooth.

4. Pour the batter into the prepared pan.

5. Put in the oven for 20 minutes.

NUTRITION: Calories: 82 Fat: 2.1 grams Net Carbs: 11.4 grams Protein:6.9 grams

30. The Keto Lovers "Magical" Grain-Free Granola

Preparation Time: 30 Minutes
Cooking Time: 1 Hour and 15 Minutes
Servings:

INGREDIENTS:

½ cup of raw sunflower seeds
½ cup of raw hemp hearts
½ cup of flaxseeds
¼ cup of chia seeds
Two tablespoons of Psyllium Husk powder
One tablespoon of cinnamon
Stevia
½ teaspoon of baking powder
½ teaspoon of salt
1 cup of water

DIRECTIONS:

1. Preheat your oven to 3000 F. Make sure to line a baking page with a parchment piece.

2. Take your food processor and grind all the seeds.

3. Add the dry ingredients and mix well.

4. Stir in water until fully incorporated.

5. Let the mixture sit for a while. Wait until it thickens up.

6. Spread the mixture evenly-giving a thickness of about ¼ inch.

7. Bake for 45 minutes.

8. Break apart the granola and keep baking for another 30 minutes until the pieces are crunchy.

9. Remove and allow them to cool.

NUTRITION: Calories: 292 Fat: 25 grams Net Carbs: 12 grams Protein: 8 grams

31. Keto Ice Cream

Preparation Time: 10 Minutes
Cooking Time: 3-4 Hours to Freeze
Servings: 4-5

INGREDIENTS:
1 ½ teaspoon of natural vanilla extract
1/8 teaspoon of salt
1/3 cup of erythritol
2 cups of artificial coconut milk, full fat

DIRECTIONS:
1. Stir together the vanilla extract, salt, sweetener, and milk.
2. If you do not come up with an ice cream machine, freeze the mixture in ice cube trays, then use a high-speed blender to blend the frozen cubes or thaw them enough to meld in a regular blender or food processor.

3. If you have an ice cream machine, just blend according to the manufacturer's directions.

4. Eat as it is or freeze for a firmer texture.

NUTRITION: Calories: 184 Fat: 19.1 grams Net Carbs: 4.4 grams Protein: 1.8 grams

32. Apple Mix

Preparation Time: 10 Minutes
Cooking Time: 4 Hours
Servings: 6

INGREDIENTS:

Six apples, cored, peeled, and sliced
1½ cups almond flour
Cooking spray
1 cup of coconut sugar
One tablespoon cinnamon powder
¾ cup cashew butter, melted

DIRECTIONS:

1. Add apple slices to your slow cooker after you have greased it with cooking spray.

2. Add flour, sugar, cinnamon, and coconut butter, stir gently, cover, cook on High for 4 hours, divide into bowls and serve cold.

NUTRITION: Calories: 200 Fat: 5 grams Net Carbs: 8 grams Protein: 4 grams

33. Almond Butter Fudge

Preparation Time: 17 Minutes

Cooking Time: 2-3 Hours to Freeze

Servings: 8

INGREDIENTS:

2 ½ tablespoons coconut oil

2 ½ tablespoons honey

½ cup almond butter

DIRECTIONS:

1. In a saucepan, pour almond butter then add coconut oil warm for 2 minutes or until melted.
2. Add honey and stir.

3. Pour the mixture into a candy container and store it in the fridge until set.

NUTRITION: Calories: 63 Fat: 4.8 grams Net Carbs: 5.6 grams Protein: 0.2 grams

34. The Vegan Pumpkin Spicy Fat Bombs

Preparation Time: 20 Minutes

Cooking Time: 1 Hour and 20 Minutes

Servings: 12

INGREDIENTS:

¾ cup of pumpkin puree

¼ cup of hemp seeds

½ cup of coconut oil

Two teaspoons of pumpkin pie spice

One teaspoon of vanilla extract

Liquid Stevia

DIRECTIONS:

1. Take a blender and add together all the ingredients.

2. Blend them well and portion the mixture out into silicon molds.

3. Allow them to chill and enjoy!

NUTRITION: Calories: 103 Fat: 10 grams Net Carbs: 2 grams Protein: 1 gram

35 Orange Cake

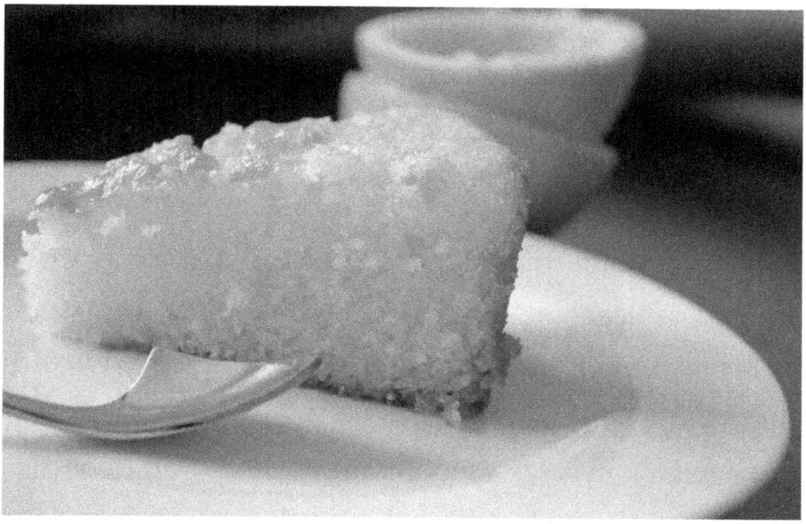

Preparation Time: 25 Minutes

Cooking Time: 5 Hours and 10 Minutes

Servings: 4

INGREDIENTS:

Cooking spray

One teaspoon baking powder

1 cup almond flour

1 cup of coconut sugar

½ teaspoon cinnamon powder

Three tablespoons coconut oil, melted

½ cup almond milk

½ cup pecans, chopped

¾ cup of water

½ cup raisins

½ cup orange peel, grated

¾ cup of orange juice

DIRECTIONS:

1. In a bowl, mix flour with half of the sugar, baking powder, cinnamon, two tablespoons oil, milk, pecans, and raisins, stir and pour this in your slow cooker after you have sprayed it with cooking spray.
2. Warm a small pan over medium heat. Add water, orange juice, orange peel, the rest of the oil, and the remainder of the sugar, stir, bring to a boil, pour over the blend in the slow cooker, cover, and cook on Low for 5 hours.

3. Divide into dessert bowls and serve cold.

NUTRITION: Calories: 182 Fat: 3 grams Net Carbs: 4 grams Protein: 3 grams

36. Chia Raspberry Pudding

Preparation Time: 10 Minutes

Cooking Time: 3 Hours

Servings: 2

INGREDIENTS:

Four tablespoons chia seeds

½ cup raspberries

1 cup of coconut milk

DIRECTIONS:

1. Add the raspberry and coconut milk into your blender and blend until smooth.

2. Pour the mixture into a mason jar.

3. Add chia seeds and stir.

4. Cap jar and shake.

5. Set in the fridge for 3 hours.

NUTRITION: Calories: 408 Fat: 38.8 grams Net Carbs: 22.3 grams Protein: 9.1 grams

37. Pumpkin Cake

Preparation Time: 20 Minutes

Cooking Time: 2 Hours and 10 Minutes

Servings: 10

INGREDIENTS:

1 ½ teaspoons baking powder

Cooking spray

1 cup pumpkin puree

2 cups almond flour

½ teaspoon baking soda

1 ½ teaspoons cinnamon, ground

¼ teaspoon ginger, ground

One tablespoon coconut oil, melted

One tablespoon flaxseed mixed with two tablespoons water

One tablespoon vanilla extract

1/3 cup maple syrup

One teaspoon lemon juice

DIRECTIONS:

1. In a bowl, flour with baking powder, baking soda, cinnamon, and ginger, then stir.

2. Add flaxseed, coconut oil, and vanilla, pumpkin puree, and maple syrup, and lemon juice, stir and pour in your slow cooker after spraying it with cooking spray parchment paper.

3. Cover Up pot and cook on Low for 2 hours and 20 minutes.

4. Leave the cake to cool down, slice, and serve.

NUTRITION: Calories: 182 Fat: 3 grams Net Carbs: 3 grams Protein: 1 gram

38. Apple Crisp

Preparation Time: 10 Minutes

Cooking Time: 40 Minutes

Servings: 6

INGREDIENTS:

½ cup vegan butter

Six large apples, diced large

1 cup dried cranberries

Two tablespoons granulated sugar

Two teaspoons ground cinnamon, divided

¼ teaspoon ground nutmeg

¼ teaspoon ground ginger

Two teaspoons lemon juice

1 cup all-purpose flour

1 cup rolled oats

1 cup brown sugar

¼ teaspoon salt

DIRECTIONS:

1. Preheat the oven to 350°F. Gently grease an 8-inch square baking dish with butter or cooking spray.

2. Make the filling. Combine the apples, cranberries, granulated sugar, a teaspoon of cinnamon, nutmeg, ginger and lemon juice

in a large bowl. Toss to coat. Move the apple mixture to the prepared baking dish.

3. Make the topping. In the same large bowl, now empty, combine the all-purpose flour, oats, brown sugar, and salt. Stir to combine. Add Up the butter and, using a pastry cutter (or two knives moving in a crisscross pattern), cut back the butter into the flour and oat mixture until the butter is small.

4. Spread the topping over the apples evenly, patting down slightly— Bake for 35 minutes or until golden and bubbly.

NUTRITION: Calories: 488 Total Fat: 9 G Carbs: 101 G Fiber: 10 G Protein: 5 G Calcium: 50 Mg Vitamin D: 0 Mcg Vitamin B12: 0 Mcg Iron: 2 Mg Zinc: 1 Mg

39. Secret Ingredient Chocolate Brownies

Preparation Time: 10 Minutes

Cooking Time: 35 Minutes

Servings: 6 to 8

INGREDIENTS:

¾ cup flour

¼ teaspoon baking soda

¼ teaspoon salt

⅓ Cup vegan butter

¾ cup of sugar

Two tablespoon water

1¼ cups semi-sweet or dark dairy-free chocolate chips

Six tablespoons aquafaba, divided

One teaspoon vanilla extract

DIRECTIONS:

1. Preheat the oven to 325°F. Line Up a 9-inch square baking pan with parchment or grease well.

2. In a large bowl, combine the flour, baking soda, and salt. Set aside.

3. In a medium saucepan, mix up the butter, sugar, and water. Bring to a boil, stirring occasionally. Reduce from heat and stir in the chocolate chips.

4. Whisk in 3 tablespoons of aquafaba until thoroughly combined. Add the vanilla extract and the remaining three tablespoons of aquafaba, and whisk until mixed.

5. Apply the mixture of chocolate to the mixture of flour and whisk until it is combined. Into the prepared tub, pour down in an even layer. Bake till the top is set for 35 minutes, but when slightly shaken, the brownie jiggles. Enable 45 minutes to 1 hour to cool completely, before removing and serving.

NUTRITION: Calories: 369 Total Fat: 19 G Carbs: 48 G Fiber: 1 G Protein:4 G Calcium: 1 Mg Vitamin D: 0 Mcg Vitamin B12: 0 Mcg Iron: 1 Mg Zinc:0 Mg

40. Chocolate Chip Pecan Cookies

Preparation Time: 10 Minutes

Cooking Time: 16 Minutes

Servings: 30 Small Cookies

INGREDIENTS:

¾ cup pecan halves, toasted

1 cup vegan butter

½ teaspoon salt

½ cup powdered sugar

Two teaspoons vanilla extract

2 cups all-purpose flour

1 cup mini dairy-free chocolate chips

DIRECTIONS:

1. Preheat the oven to 350°F. Line a large rimmed baking page with parchment paper.

2. In a small skillet over medium heat, toast the pecans until warm and fragrant, about 2 minutes. Remove from the pan. Once these are cool, chop them into small pieces.

3. Make use of an electric hand mixer or a stand mixer fitted with a paddle attachment, combine the butter, salt, and powdered sugar, and cream together on high speed for 3 to 4

minutes, until light and fluffy. Stir in the vanilla extract, then beat for 1 minute or so. Turn the mixer on low and slowly add the flour, ½ cup at a time, until a dough form. Combine the chocolate chips and pecans and mix until just incorporated.

4. Using your hands, a large spoon, or a 1-inch ice cream scoop, drop 1-inch balls of dough on the baking sheet, spread out 1 inch apart. Gently press down on the cookies to flatten them slightly. Bake for 10 to 15 minutes. Wait until just yellow around the edges. Let it cool for 5 minutes.

5. Transfer them to a wire rack. Serve or store in an airtight container.

NUTRITION: Calories: 152 Total Fat: 11 G Carbs: 13 G Fiber: 1 G Protein:2 G Calcium: 2 Mg Vitamin D: 0 Mcg Vitamin B12: 0 Mcg Iron: 0 Mg Zinc:0 Mg

41. No-Bake Chocolate Coconut Energy Balls

Period of Preparation: 15 Minutes

Cooking Time: 3 to 4 Chilling Hours**Servings:** 9 Energy Balls

INGREDIENTS:

¼ cup dry roasted or raw pumpkin seeds ¼ cup dry roasted or raw sunflower seeds ½ cup unsweetened shredded coconut Two tablespoons chia seeds ¼ teaspoon salt

1½ tablespoons Dutch-process cocoa powder ¼ cup rolled oats

Two tablespoons coconut oil, melted

Six pitted dates

Two tablespoons all-natural almond butter

DIRECTIONS:

1. Mix the pumpkin seeds, sunflower seeds, coconut, chia seeds, salt, cocoa powder, and oats in a food processor. Pulse until the mix is coarsely crumbled.

2. Add the coconut oil, dates, and almond butter. Pulse until the mixture is fused and sticks together when squeezed between your fingers.

3. Scoop out two tablespoons of the mix at a time and roll them into 1½-inch balls with your hands. Place them spaced apart on a freezer-safe plate and freeze for 15 minutes. Remove from the

freezer and keep refrigerated in an airtight container for up to 4 days.

NUTRITION: Calories: 230 Total Fat: 12 G Carbs: 27 G Fiber: 5 G Protein:5 G

42. Blueberry Hand Pies

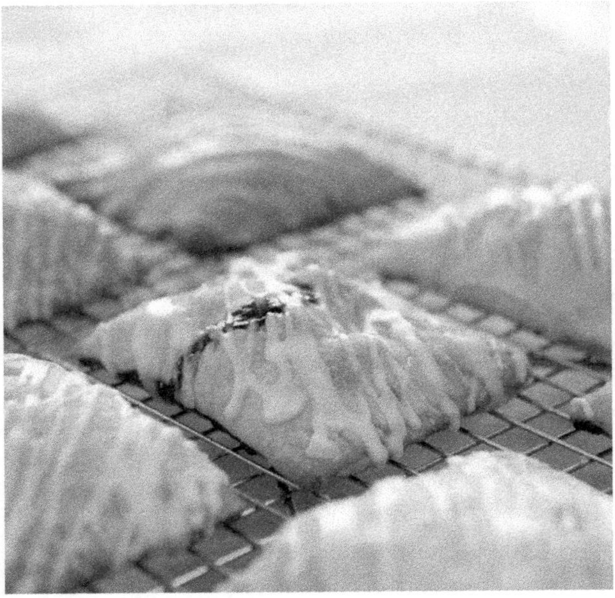

Preparation Time: 6 to 8 Minutes

Cooking Time: 20 Minutes plus Chill Time

Servings: 6 to 8

INGREDIENTS:

3 cups all-purpose flour, plus extra for sifting work surface ½ teaspoon salt

¼ cup, plus two tablespoons granulated sugar, divided

1 cup vegan butter

½ cup of cold water

1 cup fresh blueberries

Two teaspoons lemon zest

Two teaspoons lemon juice

¼ teaspoon ground cinnamon

One teaspoon cornstarch

¼ cup unsweetened soy milk

Coarse sugar, for sprinkling

DIRECTIONS:

1. Preheat the oven to 375°F. Set aside.

2. In a large bowl, merge the flour, salt, two tablespoons of granulated sugar, and vegan butter. Using a pastry cutter or two knives moving in a crisscross pattern, cut the butter into the other ingredients until the butter is small peas.

3. Add the cold water and knead to form a dough. Tear the dough in half and wrap the halves separately in plastic wrap. Refrigerate for 15 minutes.

4. Make the blueberry filling. In a medium bowl, mix the blueberries, lemon zest, lemon juice, cinnamon, cornstarch, and the remaining ¼ cup of sugar.

5. Remove one half of the dough. On a floured side, roll out the dough to ¼- to ½-inch thickness. Turn a 5-inch bowl upside down, and, using it as a guide, cut the dough into circles to make

mini pie crusts. Reroll scrap dough to cut out more circles. Repeat with the second half of the dough. You should come to an end up with 8 to 10 circles. Place the circles on the prepared sheet pan.

6. Spoon 1½ tablespoons of blueberry filling onto each circle, leaving a ¼-inch border and folding the circles in half to cover the filling, forming a half-moon shape. Use a fork to press the edges of the dough to seal the pies.

7. When all the pies are assembled, use a paring knife to score the pies by cutting three lines through the top crusts. Brush each pie with soy milk and sprinkle with coarse sugar. Bake for 20 minutes or until the filling is bubbly and the tops are golden. Let cool before serving.

NUTRITION: Calories: 416 Total Fat: 23 G Carbs: 46 G Fiber: 5 G Protein: 6 G

43. Date Squares

Preparation Time: 20 Minutes

Cooking Time: 25 Minutes

Servings: 12

INGREDIENTS:

Cooking spray, for greasing

1½ cups rolled oats

1½ cups all-purpose flour

¾ cup, plus ⅓ cup brown sugar, divided

½ teaspoon ground cinnamon

¼ teaspoon ground nutmeg

One teaspoon baking soda

¼ teaspoon salt

¾ cup vegan butter

18 pitted dates

One teaspoon lemon zest

One teaspoon lemon juice

1 cup of water

DIRECTIONS:

1. Preheat the oven to 350°F. Lightly grease or shower an 8-inch square baking plate. Set aside.

2. Make the base and topping mixture. In a large bowl, blend the rolled oats, flour, and ¾ cup of brown sugar, cinnamon, nutmeg, baking soda, and salt. Combine the butter and, using a pastry cutter or two knives working in a crisscross motion, cut the butter into the blend to form a crumbly dough. Press half of the dough into the prepared baking dish and set the remaining half aside.

3. To make a date filling, place a small saucepan over medium heat. Add the dates, the remaining ⅓ cup of sugar, the lemon zest, lemon juice, and water. Bring to a boil and cook for 7 to 10 minutes, until thickened.

4. When cooked, pour the date mixture over the dough base in the baking dish and top with the remaining crumb dough. Gently press down and spread evenly to cover all the filling. Bake for 25 minutes until lightly golden on top. Cool before serving. Store in an airtight container.

NUTRITION: Calories: 443 Total Fat: 12 G Carbs: 81 G Fiber: 7 G Protein:5 G

44. Homemade Chocolates with Coconut and Raisins

Preparation Time: 10 Minutes
Cooking Time: Chilling time
Servings: 20

INGREDIENTS:

1/2 cup cacao butter, melted
1/3 cup peanut butter
1/4 cup agave syrup
A pinch of grated nutmeg
A pinch of coarse salt
1/2 teaspoon vanilla extract
1 cup dried coconut, shredded
6 ounces dark chocolate, chopped
3 ounces raisins

DIRECTIONS:

1. Carefully combine all the ingredients, not including for the chocolate, in a mixing bowl.

2. Spoon the mixture into molds. Leave to set hard in a cool place.

3. Melt the dark chocolate in your microwave. Pour in the melted chocolate until the fillings are covered. Leave to set hard in a cool place.

NUTRITION: Calories: 130 Fat: 9.1g Carbs: 12.1g Protein: 1.3g

45. Easy Mocha Fudge

Preparation Time: 10 Minutes

Cooking Time: 60 Minutes

Servings: 20

INGREDIENTS:

1 cup cookies, crushed

1/2 cup almond butter

1/4 cup agave nectar

6 ounces dark chocolate, broken into chunks

One teaspoon instant coffee

A pinch of grated nutmeg

A pinch of salt

DIRECTIONS:

1. Line a large baking layer with parchment paper.

2. Melt the chocolate in your microwave and add in the remaining ingredients; stir to combine well.

3. Scrape the batter into a parchment-lined baking sheet. Put it in your freezer for a minimum of 1 hour to set.

4. Cut into squares and serve. Bon appétit!

NUTRITION: Calories: 105 Fat: 5.6g Carbs: 12.9g Protein: 1.1g

46. Almond and Chocolate Chip Bars

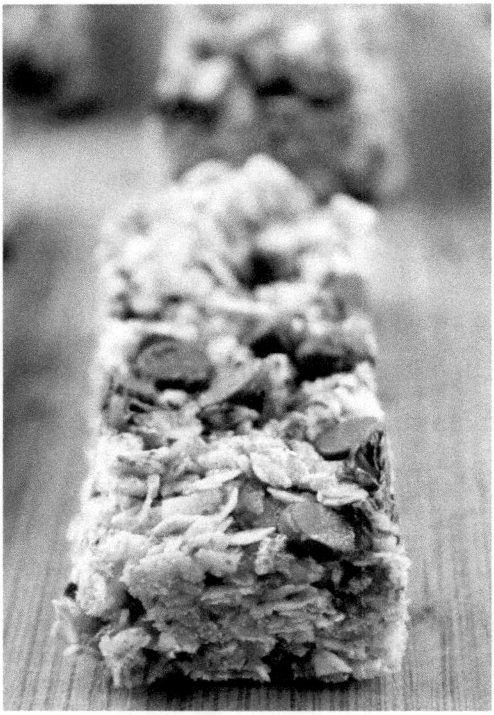

Preparation Time: 10 Minutes

Cooking Time: 30 Minutes

Servings: 10

INGREDIENTS:

1/2 cup almond butter

1/4 cup coconut oil, melted

1/4 cup agave syrup

One teaspoon vanilla extract

1/4 teaspoon sea salt

1/4 teaspoon grated nutmeg

1/2 teaspoon ground cinnamon

2 cups almond flour

1/4 cup flaxseed meal

1 cup vegan chocolate, cut into chunks

1 1/3 cups almonds, ground

Two tablespoons cacao powder

1/4 cup agave syrup

DIRECTIONS:

1. In a mixing bowl, thoroughly combine the almond butter, coconut oil, 1/4 cup of agave syrup, vanilla, salt, nutmeg, and cinnamon.

2. Gradually stir in the almond flour and flaxseed meal and stir to combine. Add in the chocolate chunks and stir again.

3. In a small blending bowl, combine the almonds, cacao powder, and agave syrup. Now, spread the ganache onto the cake. Freeze for about 30 minutes, cut into bars and serve well chilled. Enjoy!

NUTRITION: Calories: 295 Fat: 17g Carbs: 35.2g Protein: 1.7g

47. Almond Butter Cookies

Preparation Time: 10 Minutes

Cooking Time: 30 Minutes

Servings: 10

INGREDIENTS:

3/4 cup all-purpose flour

1/2 teaspoon baking soda

1/4 teaspoon kosher salt

One flax egg

1/4 cup coconut grease, at room temperature

Two tablespoons almond milk

1/2 cup brown sugar

1/2 cup almond butter

1/2 teaspoon ground cinnamon

1/2 teaspoon vanilla

DIRECTIONS:

1. In a blending bowl, blend the flour, baking soda, and salt. In another bowl, combine the flax egg, coconut oil, almond milk, sugar, almond butter, cinnamon, and vanilla. Whisk the wet mixture into the dry materials and stir until well combined.

2. Place the batter in your refrigerator for about 30 minutes. Shape the batter into small cookies and arrange them on a parchment-lined cookie pan.

3. Bake in the preheated oven at 350 degrees F for approximately 12 minutes. Later, move the pan to a wire rack to cool at room temperature. Bon appétit!

NUTRITION: Calories: 197 Fat: 15.8g Carbs: 12.5g Protein: 2.1g

48. Vanilla Halvah Fudge

Preparation Time: 10 Minutes

Cooking Time: Chilling Time

Servings: 16

INGREDIENTS:

1/2 cup cocoa butter

1/2 cup tahini

Eight dates pitted

1/4 teaspoon ground cloves

A pinch of grated nutmeg

A coarse pinch salt

One teaspoon vanilla extract

DIRECTIONS:

1. Line a square baking pot with parchment paper.

2. Mix the materials until everything is well incorporated.

3. Scrape the batter into the parchment-lined pan. Place it until it is ready for serving, in the fridge. Healthy appetite!

NUTRITION: Calories: 106 Fat: 9.8g Carbs: 4.5g Protein: 1.4g

49. Raw Chocolate Mango Pie

Preparation Time: 10 Minutes
Cooking Time: Chilling Time
Servings: 16

INGREDIENTS:

Avocado layer:
Three ripe avocados, pitted and peeled
A pinch of sea salt
A pinch of ground anise
1/2 teaspoon vanilla paste
Two tablespoons coconut milk
Five tablespoons agave syrup
1/3 cup cocoa powder
Crema layer:
1/3 cup almond butter
1/2 cup coconut cream
One medium mango, peeled
1/2 coconut flakes
Two tablespoons agave syrup

DIRECTIONS:

1. In your food processor, blend the avocado layer until smooth and uniform, reserve.

2. Then, blend the other layer in a separate bowl. Spoon the layers in a lightly oiled baking pan.

3. Transfer the cake to your freezer for about 3 hours. Store in your freezer. Bon appétit!

NUTRITION: Calories: 196 Fat: 16.8g Carbs: 14.1g Protein: 1.8g

50. Raw Raspberry Cheesecake

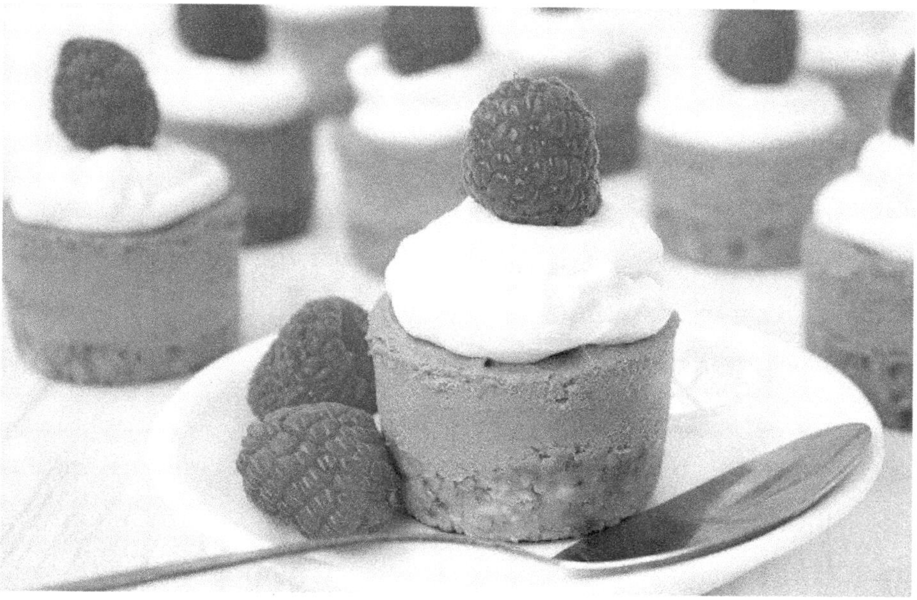

Preparation Time: 15 Minutes

Cooking Time: Chilling Time

Servings: 9

INGREDIENTS:

Crust:

2 cups almonds

1 cup fresh dates, pitted

1/4 teaspoon ground cinnamon

Filling:

2 cups raw cashews, drenched overnight and drained

14 ounces blackberries, frozen

One tablespoon fresh lime juice

1/4 teaspoon crystallized ginger

One can use coconut cream

Eight fresh dates pitted

DIRECTIONS:

1. In your food processor, blend the crust ingredients until the mixture comes together; press the crust into a lightly oiled springform pan.

2. Then, blend the filling layer until completely smooth. Spoon the filling onto the crust, creating a flat surface with a spatula. Transfer the cake to your freezer for about 3 hours. Store in your freezer. Garnish with organic citrus peel. Bon appétit!

NUTRITION: Calories: 385 Fat: 22.9 Carbs: 41.1g Protein: 10.8g